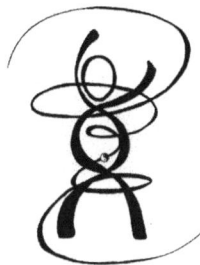

SPIRALING LIFE FORCE PRESS

Starting Your Practice

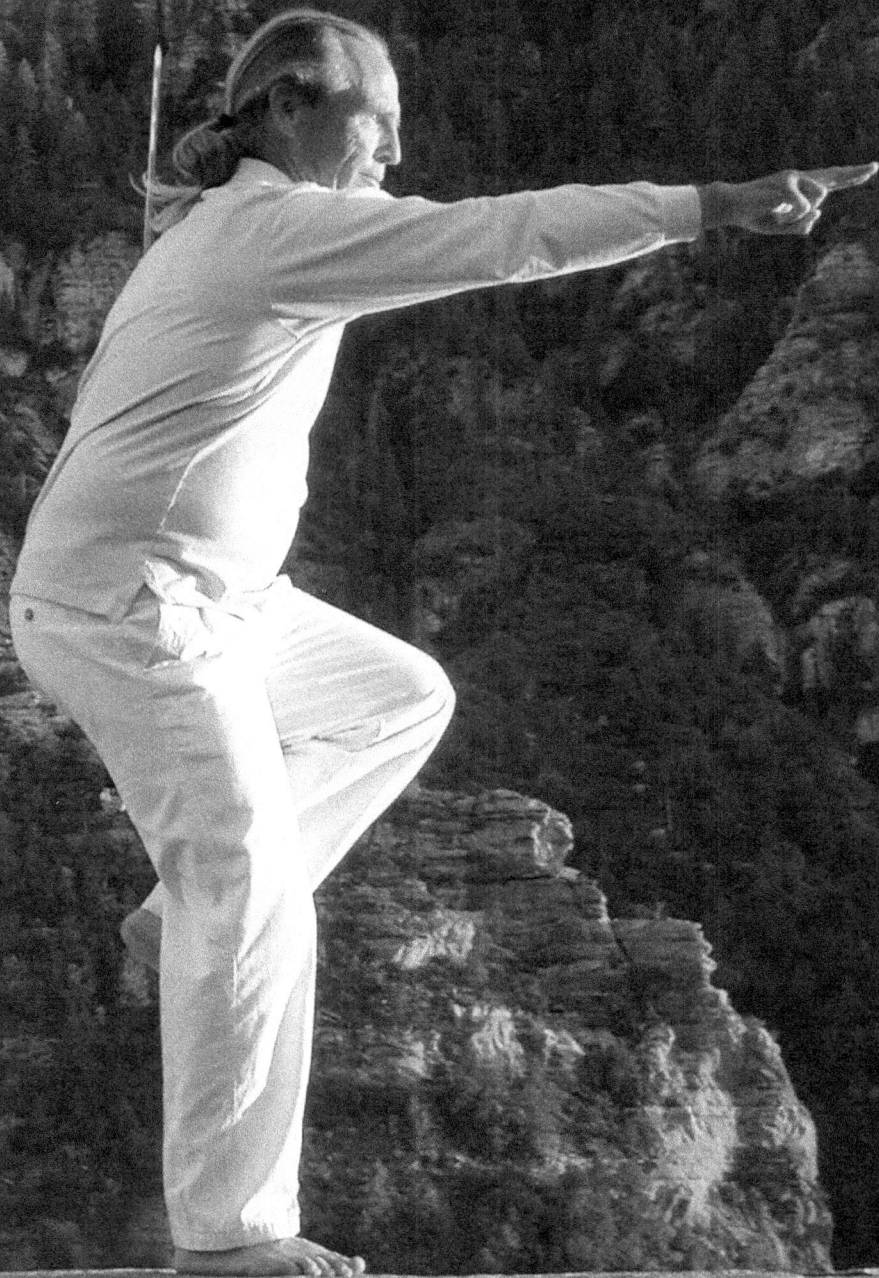

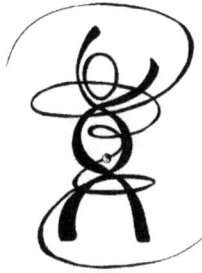

TABLE OF CONTENTS

TABLE OF CONTENTS cont.

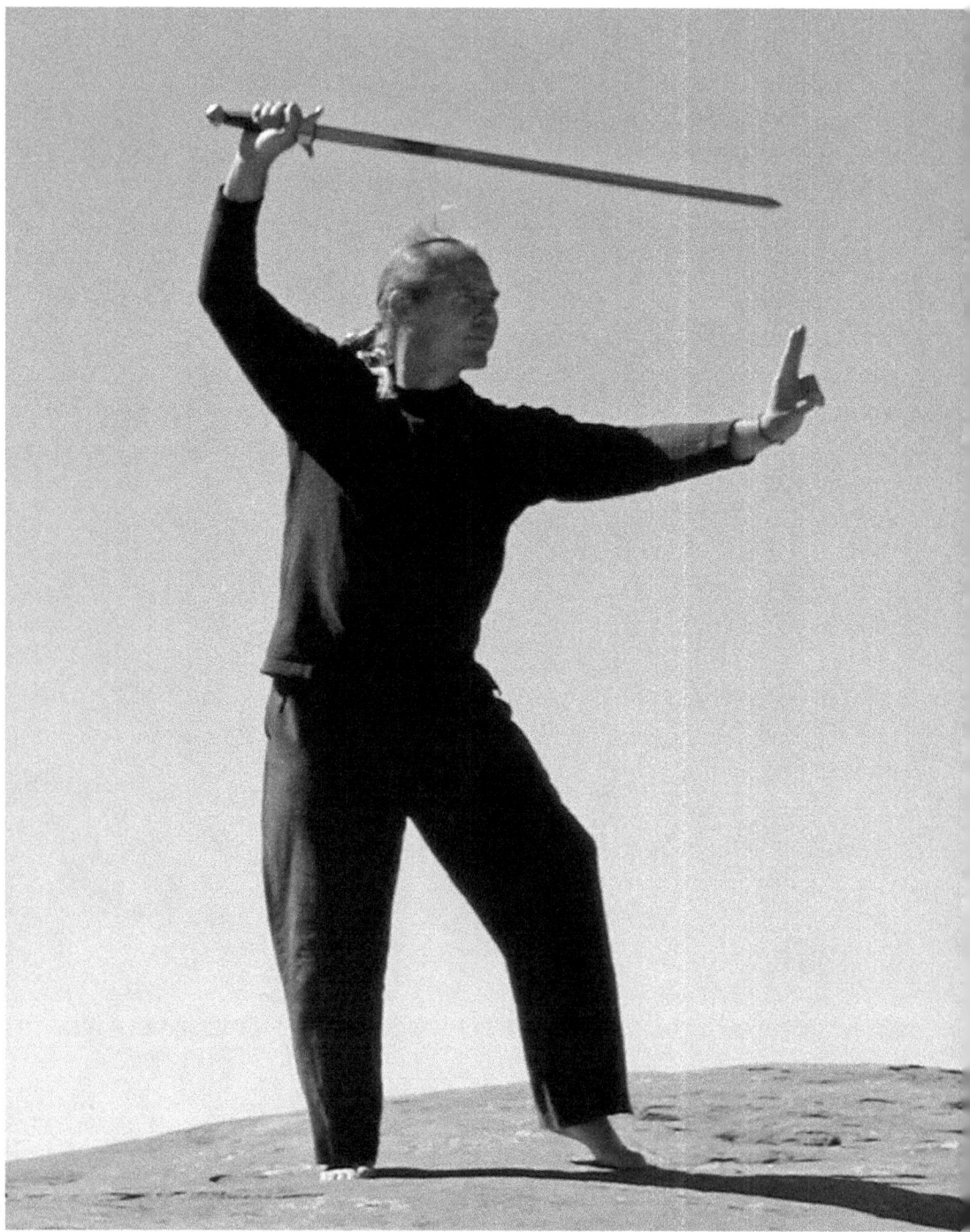

AUTHOR'S NOTE

I know that I am a student and teacher. Having said this, there are only a few things that I know, and I am just beginning to get a sense of how I know these few things. The knowing I am referring to is more than the knowing of how to do something or the knowing about something. This deeper knowing is the accepting of a belief into my consciousness as my truth. It is humbling for I am at, more or less, the midpoint of my life and really am just beginning to experience what this deep knowing is and how it works within me.

What has guided me in my life is what I can best call a feeling ~ a feeling about what truth is, and about how I as an individual can best relate to my experiences of this world. There has always been a theme running through this feeling which I now know to be oneness: the feeling of an underlying interconnectedness unifying the apparently separate things of Creation and unifying the apparently separate parts and levels within these things, including us.

Over the years, this feeling has shown me many

variations of itself: equality, inclusiveness, unlimited potential, balance, integration or harmonization, and love (the unrestricted giving and receiving or sharing between things and beings). Allowing this feeling in its many hues to interact with my daily experiences has become a valuable method for helping me decide where and with whom to invest myself, my time and energy, and for helping me choose the beliefs I will hold in my consciousness. For me, these qualities of oneness have become the hallmark of truth... they are how I recognize or know truth.

The feeling of oneness permeates Qi Gong Practice. It is what Qi Gong Practice is ~ what is taking place in one part of your body is happening in every part, and what is taking place within your physical body is simultaneously occurring in your feeling body and mental body.

The feeling of oneness is a way of knowing; it is a way of living. It is this way that I seek to share with you.

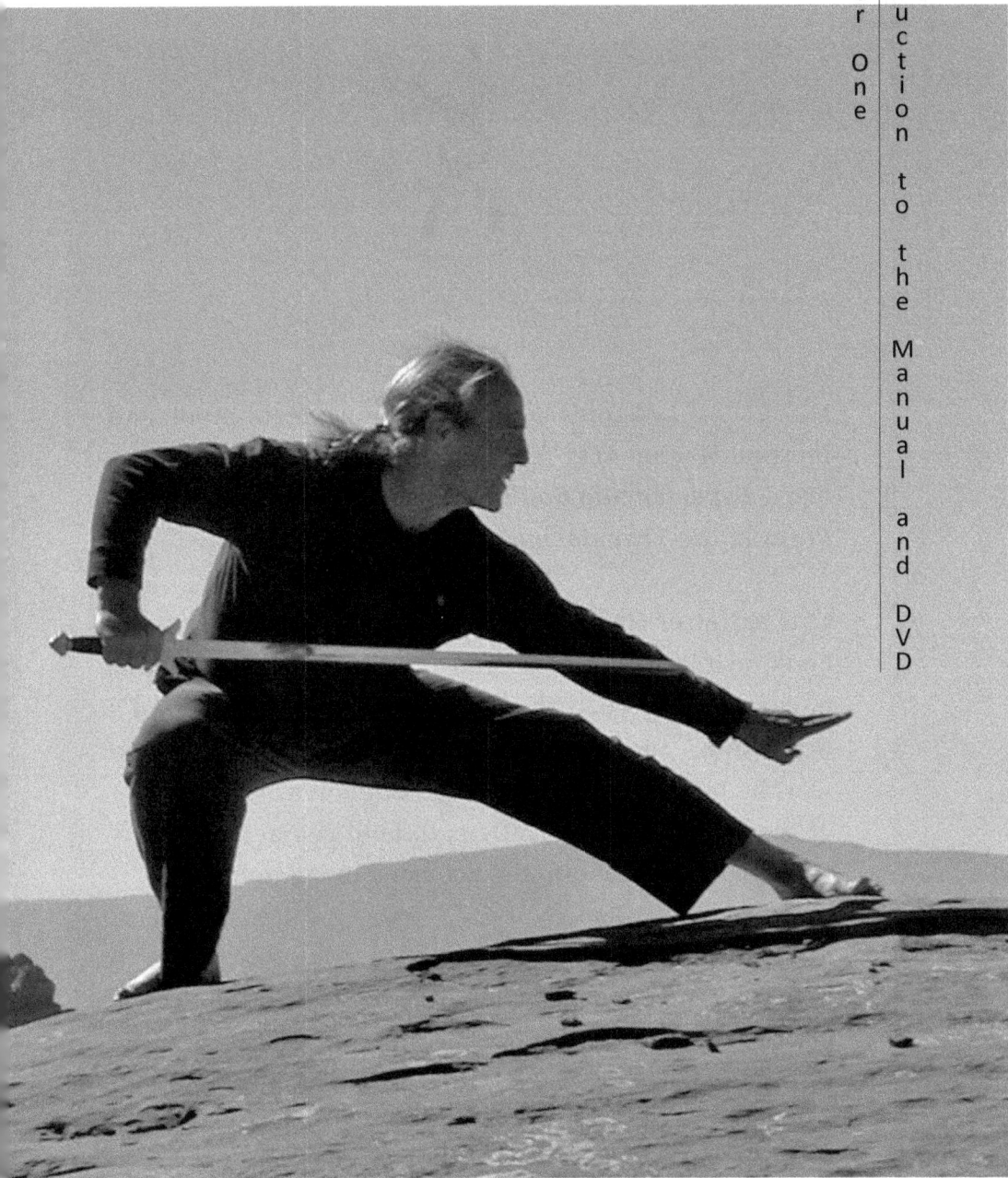

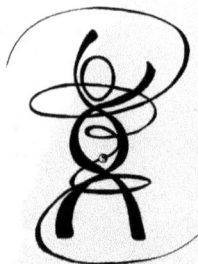

My name is Lyn Dilbeck. I am a Qi Gong, Meditation, and Internal Martial Arts Teacher, and I am the author of the book "*Experiencing God's Reflection ~ The Role Qi Gong Plays in the Transformation of Consciousness*."

This series of Manuals and DVDs is an extension of this book, so it is my hope that you are coming to this practice having already read the book. In "*Experiencing God's Reflection*," the spiritual theory of Qi Gong is shared and the methods of the practice explained. The purpose of these manuals and DVDs is to help you actualize this theory and these methods through a living practice.

Always, the primary intention of Qi Gong Practice is to help you remember Who You Are, for it is who you believe you are that guides you in choosing the beliefs, from the infinite beliefs within God, that become real to you and form your reality.

The theory of Qi Gong is the memory of Who You Are and the language by which this memory is communicated to your consciousness. What Qi Gong tells you is that you are a precious balance of God and Creation; you are both the consciousness and the being created in and from this balance. But primarily you are consciousness, the Consciousness of God, the Consciousness of Oneness and Love that is holding God, Creation, and all forms of life, together.

The method of Qi Gong Practice is how the *Keys for the Transformation of Human Consciousness* and the *Guiding Principles* are applied to your experiences of life. This is the path within you that shows you how to experience this world in a new way.

As you walk this path, you come to understand that it is you, your choice to believe that you need to judge what you experience in Creation, and your subsequent acts to control, manipulate, and own her, that keep you separate from God and limited in the expression of your will. The essence of the practice is to release these perceived needs to judge, control, and manipulate (The Essence Movement of Qi Gong Practice, ch. 13, pp 199 – 208).

In the new way, you trust and allow the divine intelligence of Creation (God Our Mother) to orchestrate her natural processes of balance and integration. You are shown how to allow the yin and yang forces of Qi that form your experiences, and that also form the altars of your mind, heart, and body (the three tan tiens), to flow into one another. This natural process forms a union of balance within each altar. Then, by way of Creations' laws of harmonics, these three altars reunify or harmonize to form your Spiritual Body. This body reflects your Soul (God within you) into Creation perfectly. It is within this spiritualized body that you, again, consciously experience the oneness and unlimited power you share with God, Creation, and your brothers and sisters (The Core Event of Qi Gong Practice, ch. 7).

All of the Guiding Principles are introduced to you in the next manual of this series, "**Guiding Principles of the Internal Arts**." But right now it is important to understand the seventh principle: *What Happens in One Tan Tien (altar) Happens in all Tan Tiens.* Here in lies the beauty and genius of Qi Gong as both a spiritual language and a path... your Soul is speaking to and guiding your consciousness through every vibrational level of Creation and your body. The Transformational Keys and Guiding Principles are equally applicable to your physical movements as they are to your experiences of emotion and thought.

Traditionally in Qi Gong, these keys and principles are first shared with a student on the Etheric Plane, the plane of energy and matter. But before you begin to study and apply the Guiding Principles to your movements, you need to form a physical foundation. This requires basic conditioning of your joints (bones, ligaments, and cartilages) and the acquisition of a number of physical skills. This manual gives you this conditioning and these skills and then codifies them within your being through a Qi Gong form ~ *The Foundation Form*.

This first manual of the series, "*Starting Your Practice*," is your invitation; it is a tangible entrance to the internal path of Qi Gong Practice.

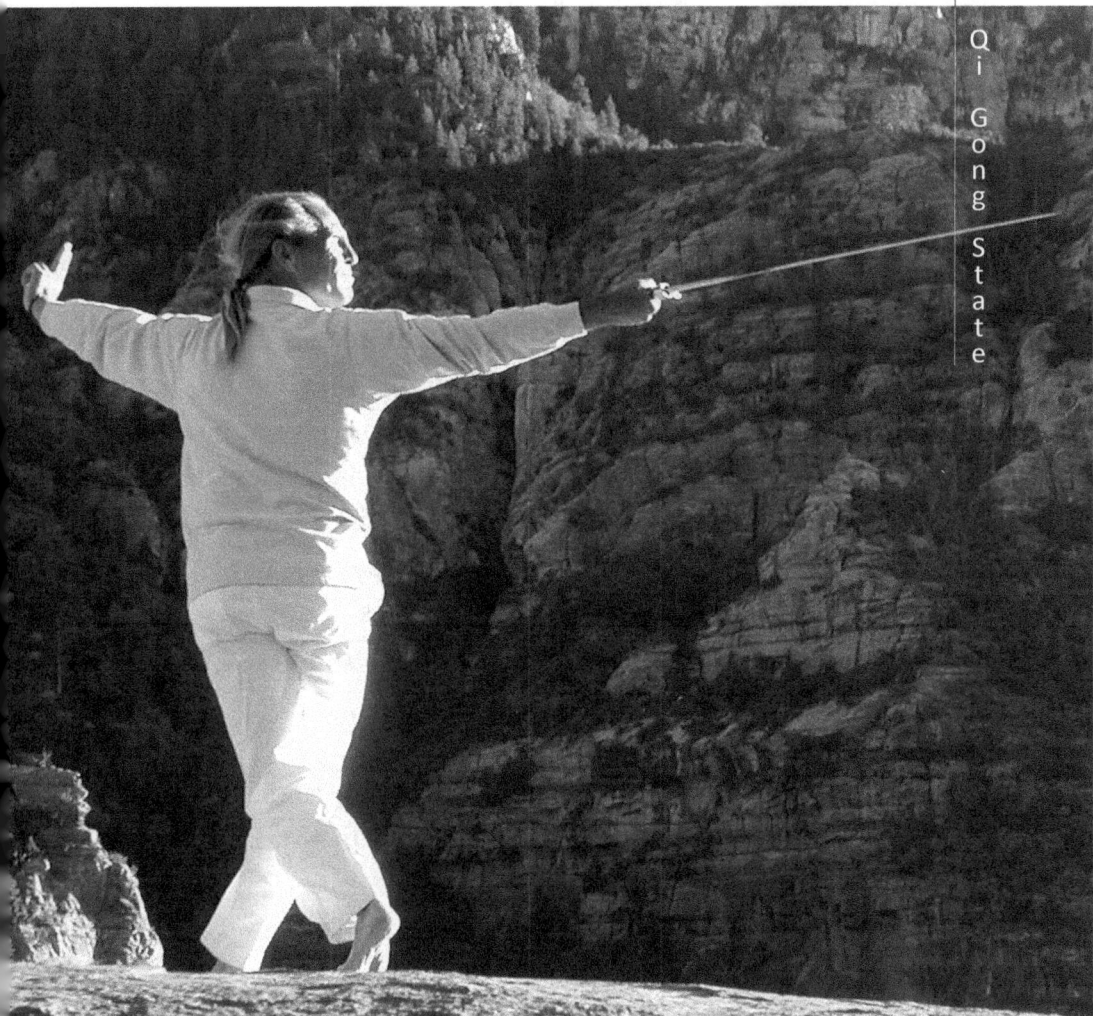

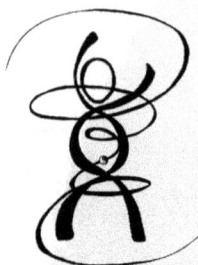

Entering the Qi Gong State ~
Your Opening Prayer

EACH SESSION OF QI GONG Practice begins by your entering the **Qi Gong State**. You may remember this from chapter 12 in the book. This means that you take a short period of time to bring your awareness, your consciousness, into the very moment you are now in ~ in other words you become present. This is how you open yourself to God, Creation (God Our Mother) and Christ. Then simply formulate your prayer.

The guidance coming through the book asks that your prayer include the following three sentiments:

- **ACCEPTANCE** of everything that has happened and is now happening in your life,
- **GRATITUDE** for all that you are, all that surrounds you, and all that is being revealed to you,

- **INVITATION** to God, Creation and Christ (all that is holy in your eyes) to participate in your life and practice.

This prayer must come from your heart and be recited with deep feeling. To serve as only an example, I share here my own prayer:

Infinite God, Creator of all, the One Spirit

Divine Goddess, God become manifest,
the divine Qi from which all of the energy, matter,
and intelligence of Creation arise.

And Christ, the holy consciousness and being,
created in the union of God Our Father
and Creation Our Mother ~
who we all are,
who the great ones are,
and who I, too, am.

I love you.
Thank you for all that I am, all that surrounds me,
and all that you are revealing to me.
I ask for your help and guidance in my life
and in the lives of all beings.

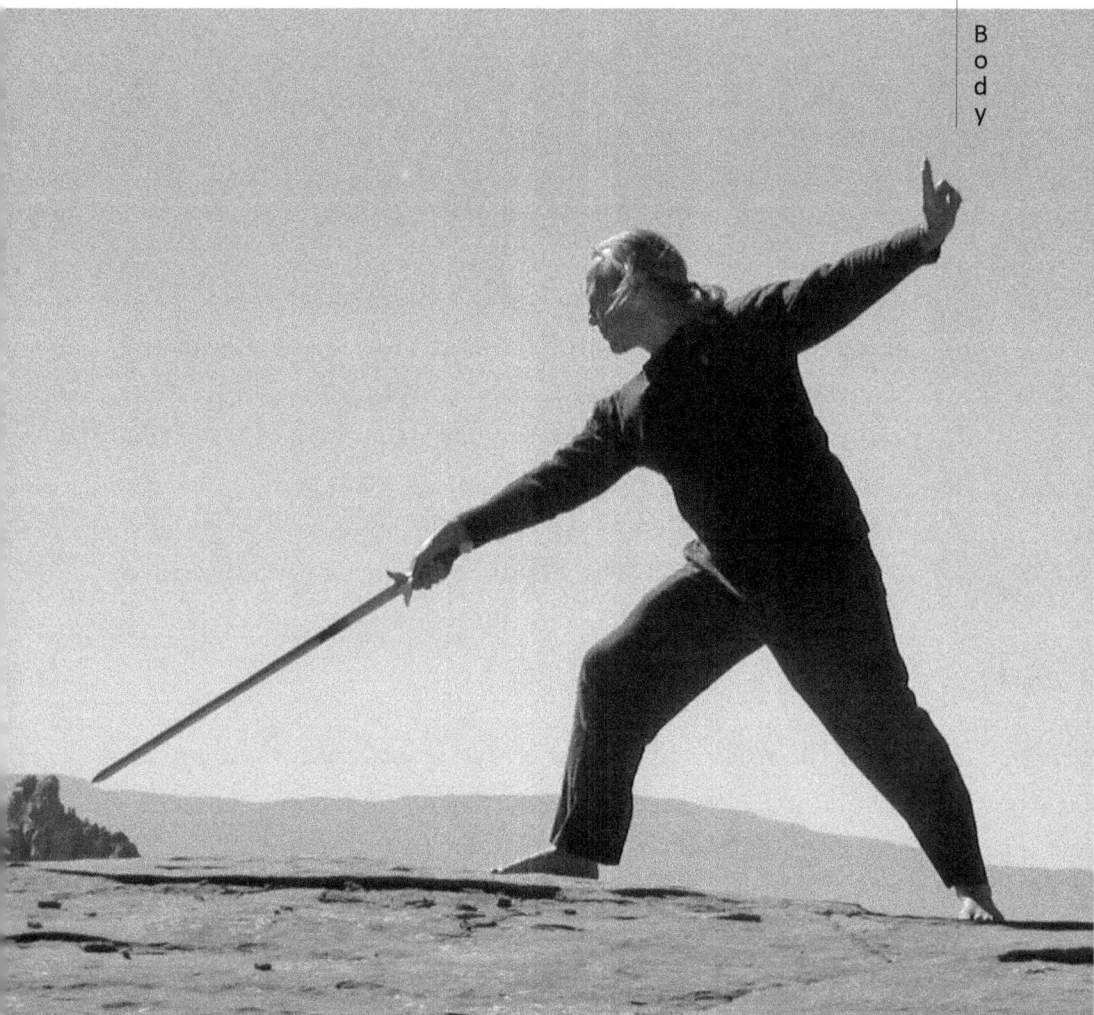

13

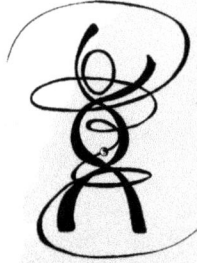

Warming Up Your Body

To BOTH FACILITATE THE FLOW of energy through your body and to avoid causing damage to your ligaments and cartilages, it is important to warm up your joints. Your joints function much like a transfer station joining one part of your body to another. And on the level of Qi, the joints transfer the energy flowing in one section of your body onto the next. The major joints are your ankles and knees, hips and pelvis, shoulders – elbows – wrists, and your spine and neck.

Start the warm-up of your body at your ankles and knees.

Circling the Knees Together

• Put your feet together with your toes pointing forward.

• Slightly bend your knees and fold at your hips to place

your hands on your knees. Relax your lower back and buttocks to release the sacral area and tailbone, while at the same time extending up through your spine to keep your head and neck erect.

• As you bend your knees, guide both of them together through half of a circle to reach the forward point on that circle. Do not drive the knees past the tips of your toes.

• As you straighten your knees, guide them through the other half of the circle, which draws both knees back in to complete the circle.

• Use the power of your sink to drive your knees through the forward arc. And use the power of your rise to draw them through the return arc.

• Do nine circles in both directions.

Circling the Knees Apart

• Now separate your feet to shoulder width, toes pointing forward.

• As you bend your knees, they will move apart and forward as each of them travels through their separate half circles.

• As you straighten your knees, they will approach one another and be drawn back in as each of them completes their circles. Again, use the power of your sink to drive the knees apart and forward, and the power of your rise to draw them toward one another and back in.

- Do nine circles.

- Then change directions. This time as you bend your knees, they will approach one another and move forward as you guide them to the front points of their separate circles. As you straighten your knees, they will move away from one another to then be drawn back in to complete their circles.

- Do nine circles.

Rocking from Ball to Heel

- Bring your feet back together.

- Your knees are slightly bent, and your hands remain on your knees. Your lower back and buttocks are still relaxed to release the sacrum and tailbone.

- As you bend your knees, rock forward onto the balls of your feet. This time you do drive your knees forward beyond the tips of your toes.

- Then, as you straighten your knees, rock back onto your heels.

- Rock forward and back nine times, making sure to do it gently.

Next, warm up your hips and pelvis.

Big Hip Circles

- Separate your feet to shoulder width, bend your knees, and place your hands on your hips.

- Keep your knees bent and your pelvis and chest facing forward as you now guide your pelvis through a large circle. First drive the pelvis forward, then to one side, to the back, to the other side, and then forward again. It is your pelvis creating this big circle; your head remains relatively still.

- Do four or five circles.

This large circle now becomes much smaller as you change to Hula Hips.

Hula Hips

- Continue to guide your pelvis through the circle. But now you will continually pull the pelvis up as you are moving through the circle by using your lower abdominal, side, and back muscles. This continual lifting as you move through the circle causes the pelvis to wobble much like a plate you have dropped on the floor.

- Do this wobbling circle nine times.

- Change directions, first doing four or five of the big circles, and then continue with nine of the Hula Hip circles.

Now warm up your shoulders and elbows.

Forward and Back Circling
of the Shoulders and Elbows

- Keep your feet shoulder width apart and place your fingertips on your chest above the breast. Your knees are slightly bent and hips slightly folded.

- As you rise, use the straightening of your knees, the extending through your spine, and the opening or expanding of your chest to lift your elbows along a path in front of your body to their highest point, and then proceed to pull them back to their furthest back position ~ the whole time keeping your finger tips on your chest.

- As you sink, use the bending of your knees, the natural contraction of your spine, and the closing or hollowing of your chest to lower your elbows along a path behind your body to their lowest and relaxed position. Remember, your fingertips remain on your chest.

- Do nine circles.

- Then reverse the direction. This time as you rise, use your straightening knees, extending spine, and opening chest to bring your elbows back and up to their furthest back position.

- As you sink, use your bending knees, contracting spine, and closing chest to lift your elbows to their highest point, and then proceed to lower them through the front path of the circle to their lowest and relaxed position.

- Do this reverse circle nine times.

Finally warm up your spine.

Head Rolling

- Stand with your feet shoulder width apart, knees slightly bent, arms relaxed at your sides.

- Now semi-relax your upper body. This means half way release the upper section of your spine, extending from your solar plexus through your neck, and half way release your head. Make sure that your shoulders and arms are completely relaxed. Your upper body is therefore semi-slumped forward.

- Very lightly push from your left foot to slightly incline your body to the right. Do not turn your body, your pelvis and chest remain forward facing. Allow your upper spine, neck, head, and shoulders to roll to the right. Then slightly incline your body back, allowing your upper spine, neck, head, and shoulders to roll to the back.

- Now very lightly push from your right foot to slightly incline your body to the left. Again, allow your upper spine, neck, head, and shoulders to roll to the left. Then slightly incline your body forward, allowing the upper spine, neck, head, and shoulders to roll forward.

- Feel this rolling action pass downward through your body to the bottoms of your feet.

- Do nine circles to the right, and then nine circles to the left.

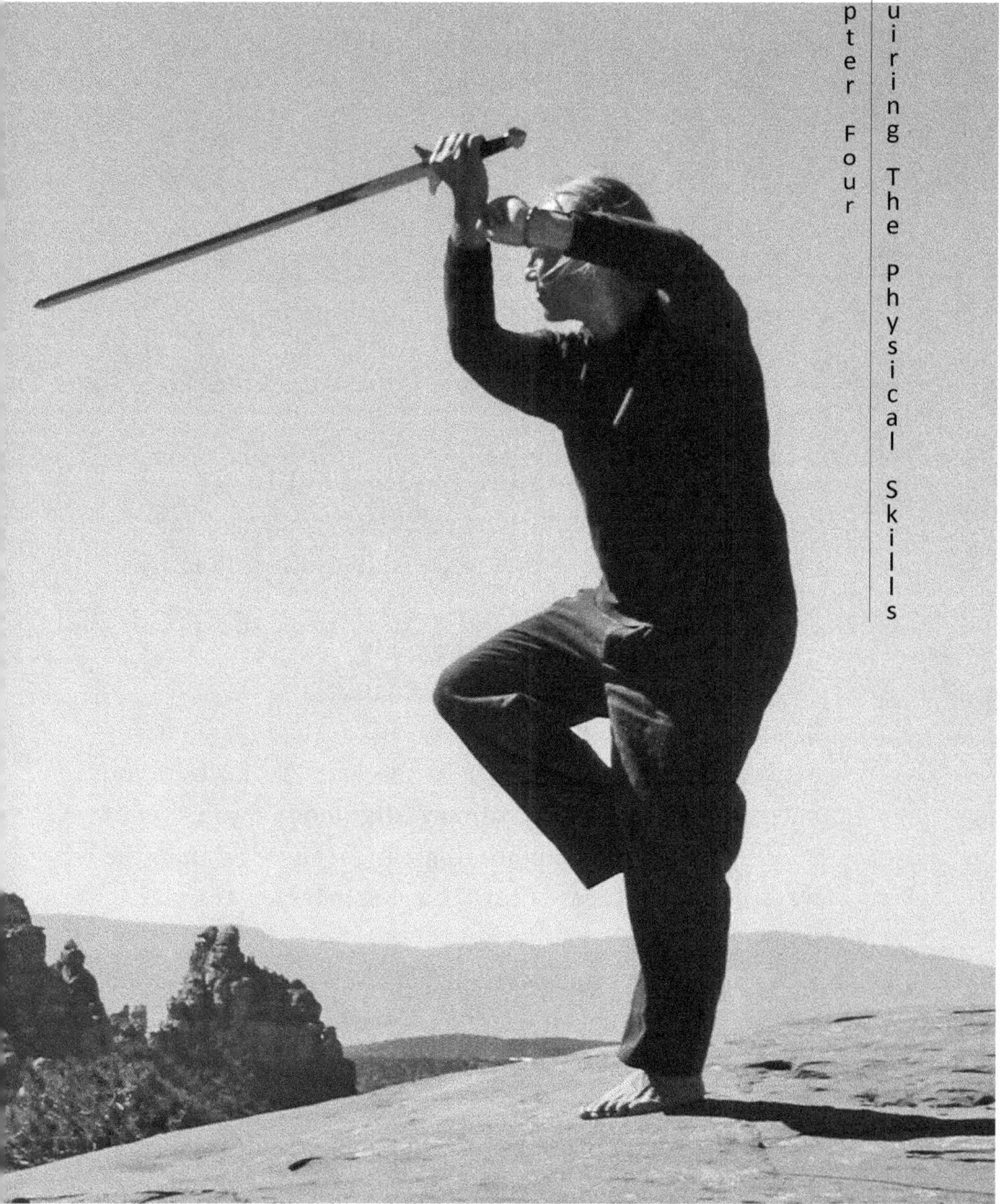

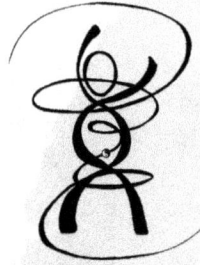

Acquiring the Physical Skills

THESE ARE THE FUNDAMENTAL SKILLS you need for the physical/energetic or etheric level of Qi Gong Practice.

The first skill is

The Standing Posture

In the **Standing Posture**, you are forming an energy bridge between the earth and the sky. To do this you must first create a **preliminary alignment** through your body, much like straightening out a hose so that the water (and in this case the Qi) can begin to flow through it.

- Open your legs and feet so that they are slightly wider than your shoulders, your knees are not locked, and your toes point straight ahead.

The **preliminary alignment** consists of **six adjustments:**
- In the **first adjustment** use "imaginative feeling" to

24

lightly pull up on a string that attaches at your crown – this point is where a line connecting the tops of both ears would pass over the top of your head. In acupuncture this point is called Bai Hui.

- For the **second adjustment**, while still pulling up on your string, bring your chin slightly down and slightly toward you. The feeling here is like the tip of your chin is making an energy connection to your Adam's apple.

- The **third adjustment** is called *Sink-Fold-Release* and consists of **three parts**. It is an important adjustment because it allows the Qi in your spine to communicate with the Qi in your legs.

The first part is to sink by slightly bending your knees.

The second part is to fold at your hips. This folding is not a pelvic tuck. Simply feel as though a bar is pressing in against your hips to slightly fold you.
At this point you feel like you are slightly bent forward in your trunk and that your tail is poking out behind.

The third part is to release your tail. Take your awareness into your lower back, sacrum, and tailbone and allow them to melt into the earth. This is a deep release of your sacral area.
At this point your tailbone feels like it is dangling from the end of your spine while at the same time your spine feels like it is extending upward.

- In the **fourth adjustment**, slightly separate your knees, as though you were straddling a horse. Do this just enough to become aware of the outside surfaces of your legs and feet.

- The **fifth adjustment** is simply to make sure that your knees are slightly bent. How much you bend your knees is completely up to you. It need not be a lot!

- And finally for the **sixth adjustment**, slightly curl your toes in order to grab the earth.

As you run through these six preliminary adjustments:
    — pull on the string
    — bring your chin down and in
    — sink-fold-release
    — separate your knees
    — make sure your knees are bent
    — and grab the earth with your toes
you are opening a channel that runs from the top of your head through your neck, spine, sacrum, tailbone and legs to the bottoms of your feet. It is in this channel that you will now experience the yin and the yang expressions of Qi.

Feel the Yin Force

In our physical-energetic world, the yin Qi expresses as a sinking and contracting force. It is energy and matter returning to a center. In the standing posture, you experience yin as energy moving down through you on its way to the center of the earth.

- To feel this, do not loose your adjustments as you completely release all of your internal organs ~ your brain, lungs and heart, all of your abdominal organs (liver, spleen, stomach, intestines, kidneys, and bladder), and release your pelvic floor. This should feel like a waterfall pouring through you into the earth. You also feel very heavy upon the earth.

Feel the Yang Force

The yang Qi expresses as a rising and expanding force. It is energy and matter moving outward away from a center. In the Standing Posture, you experience yang as energy moving up through you on its way to the sky.

- To feel this, do not lose your alignment and do not lose your feeling of the yin (the internal heaviness of your released organs and the waterfall passing down through you) as you extend your spine upward through the top of your head. This is a literal lengthening of your spine. This should feel like a geyser shooting up through you into the heavens!

- The last thing is to allow the upward moving yang force to lift your tongue. Slightly curl your tongue in order to place its tip on the hard palate about a quarter of an inch behind your front teeth.

- Feel both the yin and yang forces simultaneously. The real key here is to link the two forces ~ to feel that the downward heaviness of your released organs (the yin) is causing the upward extension of your spine (the yang).

Three Arm and Hand Positions
for the Standing Posture

As you are holding the **Standing Posture** and allowing the yin and yang forces to find and maintain their balance, you can place your arms and hands in any one of these three positions:

The first position is
Draw Earth Qi

- Extend both of your arms forward and approximately 30 degrees to the sides. The hands are just below belly button height and your palms face down.

- Your elbows are in front of the body, slightly bent and relaxed. They are closer together than your wrists. It is important that the tips of your elbows are pointing down.

- Slightly flex your wrists so that your palms literally face the earth, and keep your hands aligned with your forearms.

- Lengthen and spread your fingers and thumbs in order to open your palms.

The second position is
Embracing the Qi Ball

- Extend both of your arms forward with the palms facing one another. The middle fingers are slightly below belly button height.

- Slightly bend your elbows and wrists to form a roundness, as if you are embracing the field of energy emanating out from your lower abdomen.

- Lengthen and spread your fingers and thumbs in order to open the palms. The center of each palm is now directed toward and communicating with your Lower Tan Tien (a point approximately 2 inches below your belly button).

- The tips of your two middle fingers are 8-10 inches apart and complete the circle.

And the third position is
Palms Spiraling to Earth

- With both arms just dangling down at your sides, flex your wrists so the palms are facing the earth. The wrists bend approximately 50 degrees.

- Lengthen and spread your fingers and thumbs in order to open the palms. The center of each palm is now directed towards and communicating with the earth.

- Slightly spiral both arms inward so that your extended

fingers are pointing diagonally forward toward the body's midline. You want to feel these spirals moving through your arms and shoulders, bringing about a slight separation of your shoulder blades.

Qi Pumping in the Standing Posture

One of the easiest ways to gather and fill your body with Qi is to do Qi Pumping.

- While you are in the Standing Posture and holding the Palms Spiraling to Earth position, simply start to rhythmically bounce your body up and down by bending and straightening your knees. Be gentle.

- It is essential that you do not try to move your arms and hands, but just allow the bouncing of your body to move them for you.

- You must also maintain your Standing Posture, especially the internal softness, and the release of your low back, sacrum and tailbone.

- As your open palms move up and down, feel the "wind" on your palms. It feels as if someone were blowing or puffing air on your palms. Your internal softness will draw this "wind" into your being.

- You only need to do this practice for a minute or two to have beneficial results.

The second skill is
Sinking and Rising

Doing a series of squats every day is one of the most effective movements you can do for your physical and energetic health. The vitality of your physical and energetic bodies is dependent on your connection to both heaven and earth. We, like a magnet (and like every individual thing that exists), have a north pole and a south pole, and it is in the field created from the balance of these two poles that our anatomy and physiology unfold. But in this present time, our south pole or earth connection has become weak. As a result of this weakness, all of the systems of our bodies are under great stress, especially the immune and endocrine systems.

Squats are a powerful and direct way to strengthen your connection to the earth. The pumping action inherent to squatting also drives Qi through your entire body and keeps your spine flexible.

Squatting

• Be on a flat surface and bring your feet together.

• Simply squat down as far as you can naturally go. Do not push beyond your limits. It is important to keep your knees together and keep your heels glued to the earth. I find it helpful to wrap my arms around my upper shins when I squat.

• Then use your exhale to help you rise, extending upward through your spine to your fullest height.

• Repeat this movement at least ten times, more if you like.

Awareness of Your Internal Pumps

As you are doing your squats, focus your awareness on these three internal pumps:

— the Knee-Hip Pump (the Cua)
— the Spinal Pump
— the Chest Pump

These pumps circulate Qi in and around your body and are the source of the power behind your physical movements.

The **Knee-Hip Pump** is also called the Cua Pump. The yin action of this pump is the bending of your knees and the folding at your hips that naturally occur as you sink. The yang action is the straightening of your knees and the opening or unfolding at your hips that naturally happens when you rise.

In the **Spinal Pump** the yin action is the contraction or shortening of your vertebral column that naturally occurs as you sink. The yang action is the extension or lengthening of your vertebral column that naturally happens when you rise.

The yin action of the **Chest Pump** is the closing or

hollowing of your chest with a slight lowering of the chin and a forward rolling through the shoulders that all naturally occur as you sink. The yang action is the expansion of your chest with a slight lifting of the chin and a posterior rolling through the shoulders that all naturally happen when you rise.

Whirling Arms

- You can now use the power of these three pumps to whirl your arms. To do this, you return to the Standing Posture. Separate your feet so that they are slightly wider than shoulder width, knees slightly bend, and your toes point straight ahead. Go through the six adjustments ~ string, chin tuck, sink-fold-release, separated knees, knees bent, toes grab the earth. Feel the heaviness of your relaxed internal organs pass down through your released low back, sacrum and tailbone into your feet. At the same time feel your spine lengthen through the top of your head. The tip of your tongue touches the roof of your mouth. Completely relax your arms and hands, allowing them to dangle at your sides.

- To initiate the Whirling Arms, you first sink. Bend your knees and fold at your hips until your hands are at knee height. Now rise using all three pumps. This feels like you are jumping straight up into the sky though your feet, of course, never leave the ground. As you rise, be aware of the straightening of your knees and the unfolding of your hips. Feel the lengthening of your spine and the expansion of your chest, with a slight lifting of your chin.

• The burst of upward power from these pumps will drive your relaxed and yet extended arms through an arc in front of your body that starts with your hands at your knees and finishes with your arms and hands extended above your head. At about the midpoint of this arc, your wrists will briefly cross.

• Now sink using all three pumps. This feels like you are abruptly squatting in preparation for your next jump. As you sink, be aware of the bending of your knees and the folding of your hips. Feel the shortening of your spine and the closing of your chest with a slight lowering of your chin.

• The downward draw of these pumps will pull your relaxed and yet extended arms down through an arc in back of your body that starts with your arms and hands extended above your head and ends with your hands again at your knees.

• The important thing to feel here is how the three pumps, in both their opening (yang) phase and closing (yin) phase, propel your arms. If you go fast enough, you can completely release your arms to the power of these pumps.

• You can whirl your arms in the opposite direction just as easily. Again start by sinking. Bend your knees and fold at your hips until your hands dangle at knee height.

- This time as you rise, guide your relaxed and yet extended arms upward through the arc behind your body that starts with your hands at your knees, and finishes with your arms and hands extended above your head.

- As you sink, feel the pumps pull your arms and hands down through the arc in front of your body that starts with your arms and hands extended above your head, and ends with your hands at your knees. At about the midpoint of this arc, your wrists will briefly cross.

The third skill is
Side-to-Side Movement in the Horse Stance

Your main challenge here will be to keep your sacrum and tailbone released or soft while pushing from your legs. In the energetic anatomy of your body the yang forces run primarily through your back and the outsides of your legs. The yin forces run primarily through the front of your body and the insides of your legs.

When you move your body, the yang forces increase in power, shooting upward through your legs and spine. And because the sacrum forms the point of intersection between both of your legs and your spine, it becomes maximally yang. Tremendous yang force is moving through this area during movement. This is why it is hugely important to keep this sacral area soft, especially while you are moving. The softness of yin allows the tissues to stay malleable so they can adjust to these strong flows of energy, and also allows the yin and yang forces to find their balance.

- Form a **Horse Stance**. This is simply a lower and wider version of your Standing Posture. So, assume the Standing Posture but now with a wider placement of your feet. Your knees will be a little more bent, and the deeper fold at your hips will incline your spine a bit more forward.

- Do not rise or sink as you push from your left leg. This will move your body to the right. Feel how the heaviness of your relaxed internal organs and the sustained softness within your sacral area create an opposing energetic field that the right side of your pelvis runs up against.

- Now push from your right leg. This will move your body to the left. Again feel how the heaviness of your internal organ release and the sustained softness within your sacral area create the opposing energetic field that the left side of your pelvis runs up against.

This feeling of an opposing field is called peng. Peng is an expression of Qi that occurs when the yin and yang forces of Qi flow into one another. To me, peng feels like two puffy marshmallows pressing into each other. The bouncy quality of peng is the natural power behind all of our movements from walking and jumping to the movements in dance and martial arts.

The fourth skill is

Side-to-Side Movement with Tan Tien Turning

The tan tiens are the vibrational centers within your being that permit you to exist in and experience the different levels of this reality. These three centers are the physical-energetic, feeling-emotional, and the mental aspects of your being. But these three tan tiens also occupy a physical place in your body. The Lower Tan Tien expresses as your legs and pelvis, the Middle Tan Tien as your spine and chest, and the Upper Tan Tien as your neck and head and also includes your arms and hands. It helps to think of your tan tiens as the three parts of a tree: the roots, the trunk, and the branches and leaves respectively. The spiraling or turning of these tan tiens to the left and to the right is the most powerful of your internal pumps. The actual turning to one direction is the yang action of this pump. The internal resistance that is always pulling the body back to neutral or to face forward, is the yin action.

- Start with the **Side-to-Side Movement in the Horse Stance**.

- For this exercise, keep your arms and hands completely relaxed, dangling at your sides.

- As you are pushing out of your left leg and your body is moving to the right, you will now also turn your legs and pelvis to the right to their natural stop. In the action of turning your legs and pelvis, you also are turning your spine and chest, and your neck and head.

- Then proceed to turn your spine and chest further to the right to their natural stop.

- And finally turn your neck and head to their natural stop.

- Now push out of your right leg, which is moving your body to the left. Sequentially turn your three tan tiens to the left, starting with your legs and pelvis.

- During each phase of the turning movements, remember to feel the heaviness of your internal organ release and the sustained softness within your sacral area. This heaviness and softness (yin forces) must be proportional to the effort you exert in your pushing and turning (yang forces). This will be even more challenging because the spiraling of the tan tiens is your most powerful internal pump. This twisting action is your most yang expression.

The fifth skill is
Forward and Back Movement in the Bow Stance
To do this movement, you must first learn the **Bow Stance**. This is the same stance you would use to shoot a bow or a rifle.

- This skill does not involve your arms and hands, so allow them to simply dangle at your sides.

- Start with your feet together, and then pivot your right foot on the heel so the toes point 45° to the right. Slightly bend your right knee as you place all of your weight into the right leg.

- Extend your left foot straight forward and approximately three inches to your left with your toes pointing straight forward.

- How far you extend this leg depends on the depth of your internal release into your right leg and how much you bend your right knee. There should be no weight committed to your left foot and no leaning back in your trunk to place the left foot.

- You now put 30% of your weight into your left foot to give your stance a 30% front, 70% back, weight distribution.

- Turn your body so that your pelvis, chest and head are now facing forward. Check to see that you have a three-inch channel running between your feet from front to back. This channel is important for your balance and to open the pelvic floor.

- Form the **Standing Posture** while in this new stance. Remember the six adjustments, the internal organ release, and the reciprocal extension through your spine. The tip of your tongue touches the roof of your mouth.

- Do not rise or sink and do not lean your trunk forward or backward as you push from your back right leg. This will move your body forward.

Do Not Drive Your Left Knee Beyond The Tips of Your Toes!

• Now push from your forward left leg. This will move your body back. Stop when your tailbone points straight down to your back right heel. Do not lean your trunk backward. If you cannot reach this back alignment, it is because you extended your left leg too far forward. Simply draw it in sufficiently to allow your tailbone to come into this alignment.

• Again feel how the heaviness of your internal organ release and the sustained softness within your sacral area create an opposing field that receives the yang force of your push, both in the forward and the backward movements.

• Of course, you will want to do this movement on the other side as well.

Your sixth skill is
Forward and Back Movement with Tan Tien Turning

• To start, you are in the Bow Stance with your right foot back, the toes pointing 45° to the right. Your left foot is extended forward with the toes pointing straight forward. Make sure that you have a three-inch channel running between your feet from front to back.

• When you are in the back position with your tailbone pointing down to the right heel, turn your pelvis, chest, and head to face 45° to the right.

- As you push from your back right leg and your body is moving forward, you will now, starting with your Lower Tan Tien, sequentially turn your legs and pelvis, spine and chest, and neck and head to face forward. All three levels will come to face forward just as your front left knee arrives at its stopping point.

- Then, as you push from your forward left leg and your body is moving back, you will, starting with your Lower Tan Tien, sequentially turn your legs and pelvis, spine and chest, and neck and head, to face 45° to the right. All three levels come to face the 45° direction just as your tailbone reaches its alignment with the back right heel.

- Just like in the **Side-to-Side Movement with Tan Tien Turning**, the spiraling action of your tan tiens makes it extra challenging to keep your internal organs relaxed and your sacral area soft. Focus on this in your practice. Your reward will be plenty of peng!

- Of course, you will want to switch legs to play on the other side.

The seventh skill:
The Movement Within Your Hands
The subtle opening and closing of your palms regulates the Lou Gong Point. This special point in the center of

your palms is a portal or passageway for giving and receiving Qi. As you progress in your practice, your innate ability to issue forth and draw in Qi through your Lou Gong Points will play an important part in the healing of yourself and others. This ability can also be applied in martial arts.

• While doing your practice, always use your "imaginative feeling" to direct your awareness into and through your palms and fingers. This is as much a mental intending as it is a physical action. So literally lengthen and spread your fingers and thumbs. This intention and physical act opens your palms, which in turn opens this portal.

• Your hands and fingers should not be rigid, and yet they should not be wilted or overly soft either. You need to find "your middle zone".

Breathing Palms

Breathing Palms is a powerful and effective exercise for developing the Lou Gong Points within your palms.

• Take a medium wide Horse Stance. Remember, the Horse Stance is simply a lower, wider version of the Standing Posture. So place the inside edges of your feet at approximately shoulder width. Then continue with your six adjustments ~ string, chin tuck, sink-fold-release, separated knees, knees bent, and toes grabbing the earth. Feel the heaviness of your relaxed internal organs passing down through your released sacral area into your feet. Also feel your spine lengthen through the top of your head. The tip of your tongue touches the roof of your mouth.

• Place both hands about 15 inches out in front of your body at shoulder height and width. Your palms face forward, fingers pointing up. Your elbow tips are pointing down and are in their lowest possible position.

• On your exhale, slightly sink with a relaxed sacrum and tailbone. As you are sinking, press your spreading palms with lengthening fingers and thumbs straight forward to their natural stop, the whole time keeping your wrists flexed and your elbows unlocked and pointing down.

• Direct your awareness into your spreading palms, feeling your exhale issuing forth from your Lou Gong Points. This movement feels like you are sitting down on a "whoopee cushion" and the "noise" is projecting out of your palms.

• Inhale as you rise. As you are rising, feel how your opening chest draws your arms and hands in toward your shoulders. Your hands are now six inches in front of your shoulders, your elbows are relaxed and down. Your wrists slightly release, now not so flexed, and you also slightly relax your palms, now not so spread.

• Continue to direct your awareness into your now more relaxed palms, feeling how your inhalation is being drawn in through your Lou Gong Points. In this phase of the movement your palms have softened and feel like "mini black holes" sucking everything into them.

• Repeat this movement many times ~ until you feel the breathing quality of your palms.

The eighth skill is
Integrating Your Arms and Hands with Your Body
Every movement comes out of the internal pumps of your body ~ the **knee-hip**, **spinal**, and **chest pumps** and the **pump of your turning tan tiens**. Your arms and hands receive and then express the energy that comes to them from these pumps, which also includes the spiraling motion coming into them from the tan tiens. Moving out from your spine, these spirals pass through your shoulders, elbows, and wrists to arrive in your hands.

In order to allow this energy to flow without impediments from your internal pumps to your hands, you have to keep your shoulders, elbows, and wrists relaxed, even as they are moving. Your shoulders act much like a very heavy ball rolling around in the bottom of a bowl. Your elbows, even as they are moving and transferring these spirals, must also feel heavy and down. They act much like a heavy person swinging in a hammock. And lastly, your wrists act like a willow branch, having both flexibility and strength.

In their expressions of energy, your arms and hands move much like a ribbon flowing from the end of a moving stick. In this analogy:

— Your body with its internal pumps would be the hand that moves the stick.
— Your elbows and forearms are the stick.
— Your wrists are where the ribbon attaches.
— And your hands are the flowing ribbon.

As you now incorporate your arms and hands into the basic movements you have learned, really feel this downward heaviness in your shoulders and elbows. Also feel an internal extending or lengthening through your arms, hands, and fingers without tensing them. This feeling is similar to how water flows through a hose without the hose becoming stiff. This internal extension gives your arms and hands flexibility, and at the same time, inner strength.

The overall feeling in your movements is that your body's movements pass directly into your elbows, which then lead your wrists. Your wrists in turn lead your hands. In Qi Gong Practice, this is stated as "the body leads the hands".

Sinking and Rising ~ Now with Extended Arms

• With your feet shoulder width apart and toes pointing forward, form the Standing Posture. Remember the six adjustments ~ string, chin tuck, sink-fold-release, separated knees, knees bent, toes grab the earth. Feel the heaviness of your relaxed internal organs passing down through your released low back, sacrum and tailbone into your feet. At the same time feel your spine lengthening through the top of your head. The tip of your tongue touches the roof of your mouth.

• Extend both arms forward, shoulder width, palms facing down, the tops of your wrists at breast height. Your elbows are slightly bent with the tips of your elbows pointing down. Your wrists are also relaxed.

• Employ everything you have just learned about allowing your body's energy to flow into your arms and hands. While you internally extend or lengthen through your arms, hands and fingers, really feel the downward heaviness in your shoulders and elbows, and feel the flexible strength in your wrists. Maintain this inner extension with outer relaxation while you are moving.

• Always start your movements in your feet and legs. So, on your inhale, rise by pushing against the earth. Feel your knees and hips straightening or unfolding. Feel the lengthening of your spine and the opening of your chest. Upon receiving the energy from these internal pumps, your extended arms will now be lifted three to four inches above shoulder height. Your wrists will slightly bend, allowing your hands and fingers to flow from the ends of your rising arms.

- On your exhale, sink by bending your knees and folding at your hips. Feel your spine contracting and your chest closing. Upon receiving the energy from these pumps, your extended arms will now be lowered to mid-thigh height. Your wrists will slightly flex, allowing your hands and fingers to flow from the ends of your lowering arms.

- As your arms and hands become expressions of your body's energy, another important integration takes place ~ the integration of your neck and head with your arms and hands. Your neck, head, arms and hands together actually form your Upper Tan Tien. This integration naturally occurs when you follow your hands with your eyes. So watch your hands as they are lifted and lowered by your body.

- Continue to rise and sink until you feel that your arms and hands are being moved by your body. This feeling is similar to how your legs would move long flippers.

Side-to-Side Movement with Tan Tien Turning ~ Now with Spiraling Arms

- Take a medium wide Horse Stance by placing the inside edges of your feet at approximately shoulder width. Form the Standing Posture remembering the six adjustments ~ string, chin tuck, sink-fold-release, separated knees, knees bent, toes grab the earth. Feel the heaviness of your relaxed internal organs passing down through your released low back, sacrum and tailbone into the earth.

Feel your spine lengthening through the top of your head. The tip of your tongue touches the roof of your mouth.

- Extend both arms forward at shoulder width, palms facing down, and the tops of your wrists at breast height. Your elbows are slightly bent with the tips of your elbows pointing down. Your wrists are relaxed.

- Employ again everything you have learned about allowing your body's energy to flow into your arms and hands. While you internally extend or lengthen through your arms, hands, and fingers, really feel the downward heaviness in your shoulders and elbows, and the flexibility of your wrists. Your challenge here is to maintain this inner extension with outer relaxation not only as you are moving your arms and hands, but also as you allow them to spiral.

- Remember that you always start your movements in your feet and legs. So push from your left foot, this will move your body to the right. As you are moving right, you will also turn your legs and pelvis and your spine and chest (your Lower and Middle Tan Tiens) to the right to their natural stopping points.

- Allow the push from your foot and leg and the turning of your tan tiens to move your arms and hands to the right while maintaining the shoulder width distance separating them.

- As your arms and hands move right they also spiral. Feel how the spiraling of your spine enters your shoulders, elbows, wrists, and hands to turn your palms to face right. Your right hand will travel through a 90° arc to your right side, your left follows about 15 inches behind.

- Your neck and head and your arms and hands integrate into a single movement as you follow your lead hand with your eyes. In this movement when you turn right, your right hand is the lead hand.

- At the end of your turn, both hands are horizontal, palms facing outward. Your hands and fingers are trailing behind your wrists in the same way that a ribbon would flow from the end of a moving stick. Be careful here to not lift or lower your arms and hands, they remain at chest height.

- Now push from your right foot, this will move your body to the left. As you are moving left, turn your Lower and Middle Tan Tiens (your legs and pelvis, spine and chest) to the left to their natural stopping point. Use these body movements to move your arms and hands to the left. Again feel how the spiraling of your spine enters your shoulders, elbows, wrists and hands to turn your palms to face left. Watch your lead hand. When turning left in this movement, your left is the lead hand.

- As your arms and hands complete their arc, your left hand will be extended out from the left side of your body with your right following about 15 inches behind. Both hands are horizontal, palms facing outward, hands and fingers trailing behind your wrists.

Side-to-Side Movement with Tan Tien Turning ~
Now with Spiraling Arms Forming the
Circle of Four Expressions

- Start this movement from the finishing position of the previous movement.

- You continue to be in a medium wide Horse Stance and in the Standing Posture. While still pushing from your right foot, you have turned your Lower and Middle Tan Tiens left to their natural stopping points. Both of your arms have moved left, extending out to the left side of your body at chest height. Your hands are about 15 inches apart, horizontal, palms facing outward, fingers trailing behind your wrists. You are watching your lead left hand.

- Rise slightly as you lift your arms and hands to head height while rotating both arms so that your palms face down. Maintain the 15-inch separation between your hands. Your shoulders are relaxed; your elbows are slightly bent with the tips of your elbows pointing down, and your wrists are relaxed. Feel the internal extending or lengthening through your arms, hands and fingers.

- It is easier to first learn this circular movement as a square and also allow your body to outwardly express the rise and the sink of the first three pumps. Later, the square will become a circle and there will be no rising or sinking.

- To form the left side of the square, simply sink by bending your knees and folding at your hips. Feel your spine contract and your chest close. Through the closing action of these three pumps, lower your extended arms to approximately upper thigh height. Your wrists are flexing to allow your hands and fingers to flow from the ends of your lowering arms. Your palms are facing down. Remember to watch your hands.

- To form the bottom of the square, push from your left foot to move your body to the right. At the same time turn your legs and pelvis and your spine and chest to the right to their natural stopping points. Use these body movements to both move and spiral your arms and hands across the bottom of the square. Your wrists remain slightly flexed with your hands and fingers trailing behind your wrists.

- The spirals in your arms and hands are turning your palms down and diagonally forward. Watch your lead right hand. At the end of your turn, your right hand is at the 60° right diagonal, upper thigh height, and approximately six inches out from your leg. The left is following 15 inches behind.

- To form the right side of the square, simply rise by straightening or unfolding your knees and hips, also lengthen through your spine and open your chest. Through the opening action of these three pumps, lift your extended arms to head height while gradually rotating both arms so that your palms face down. Maintain the 15-inch separation between your hands. Your shoulders are relaxed; your elbows are slightly bent with the tips of your elbows pointing down. Your wrists flex to again allow your hands and fingers to flow from the ends of your rising arms. Remember to watch your hands. At the end of this rise, the tops of your flexed wrists are even with the top of your head.

- To form the top of the square, push from your right foot to move your body to the left. At the same time turn your legs and pelvis and your spine and chest to the left to their natural stopping point. Use these body movements to both move and spiral your arms and hands across the top of the square at head height. Maintain the 15-inch separation between your hands. Your wrists remain slightly flexed with your hands and fingers trailing behind the wrists. The spirals in your arms and hands turn your palms to face forward and diagonally up. Watch your lead left hand.

- You can, of course, run through this square in the opposite direction.

In the advanced expression of this movement, you transform the square into a circle. To do this you must allow the yin and yang forces of Qi to flow into one another; you must express both at the same time. In your physical/energetic body, this happens in a couple of ways:

As you are rising (yang force) you are internally relaxing (yin force). And as you are sinking (yin force) you are at the same time feeling the upward-pushing yang force.

Another way is when you are turning your tan tiens (your legs and pelvis, spine and chest, and your neck-head-arms-hands) to the right, they are at the same time being opposed by a left spiral. And when you are turning your tan tiens to the left, they are being opposed by a right spiral.

The internal marriage of the yin and yang expressions of Qi give rise to the peng force. The Essence Movement of Qi Gong Practice (ch. 15, pp 231, 232) is to allow this internal marriage of the yin and yang. The principals that guide us, and how we apply these principals in all movement, will be discussed further in the next manual and DVD that focus on the Guiding Principals of Qi Gong Practice.

• To experience the Circle of Four Expressions, start in the left upper corner of the square. You have pushed your body to the left from your right foot, and your tan tiens are turned left. Your arms are extended to the left; the backs of your flexed wrists are head height, palms facing down.

• As you push from your left foot, feel the internal heaviness of your relaxed organs and relaxed low back, sacrum, and tailbone merge with the rise-push force of your leg. Use the resulting peng force to contract your spine and close your chest; also use the peng force to turn your tan tiens to the right. As your body is moving right and turning right, draw your spiraling arms and hands down and to the right. Watch your lead right hand. Also feel the opposing left spiral coming out of your right leg.

- As you now push from your right foot, feel again the internal heaviness of your relaxed organs and relaxed low back, sacrum and tailbone merge with the rise-push force of your leg. Use the resulting peng force to lengthen your spine and open your chest; also use it to turn your tan tiens to the left. As your body is moving left and turning left, draw your spiraling arms and hands up and to the left. Watch your lead left hand. Also feel the opposing right spiral coming out of your left leg.

- To change the direction of the circle, push from your left foot, which moves your body to the right and turns your tan tiens to the right. Use these body movements to bring your hands to the right, upper corner of the "square". At this point, your arms are extended to the right; your palms are facing down, and your extended fingers are pointing away from you to the right. The backs of your slightly flexed wrists are head height with approximately 15 inches separating them.

- To initiate the movement, now push from your right leg to move your body left, turn your tan tiens left, and draw your spiraling arms and hands down and to the left.

Before bringing this section to a close, I want to point out that the last two movements:

**Side-to-Side Movement with Tan Tien Turning ~
Now with Spiraling Arms**

and

**Side-to-Side Movement with Tan Tien Turning ~
Now with Spiraling Arms Forming the
Circle of Four Expressions**

can also be done in the Bow Stance. After mastering these skills in the Horse Stance, I invite you to do them in the Bow Stance as well.

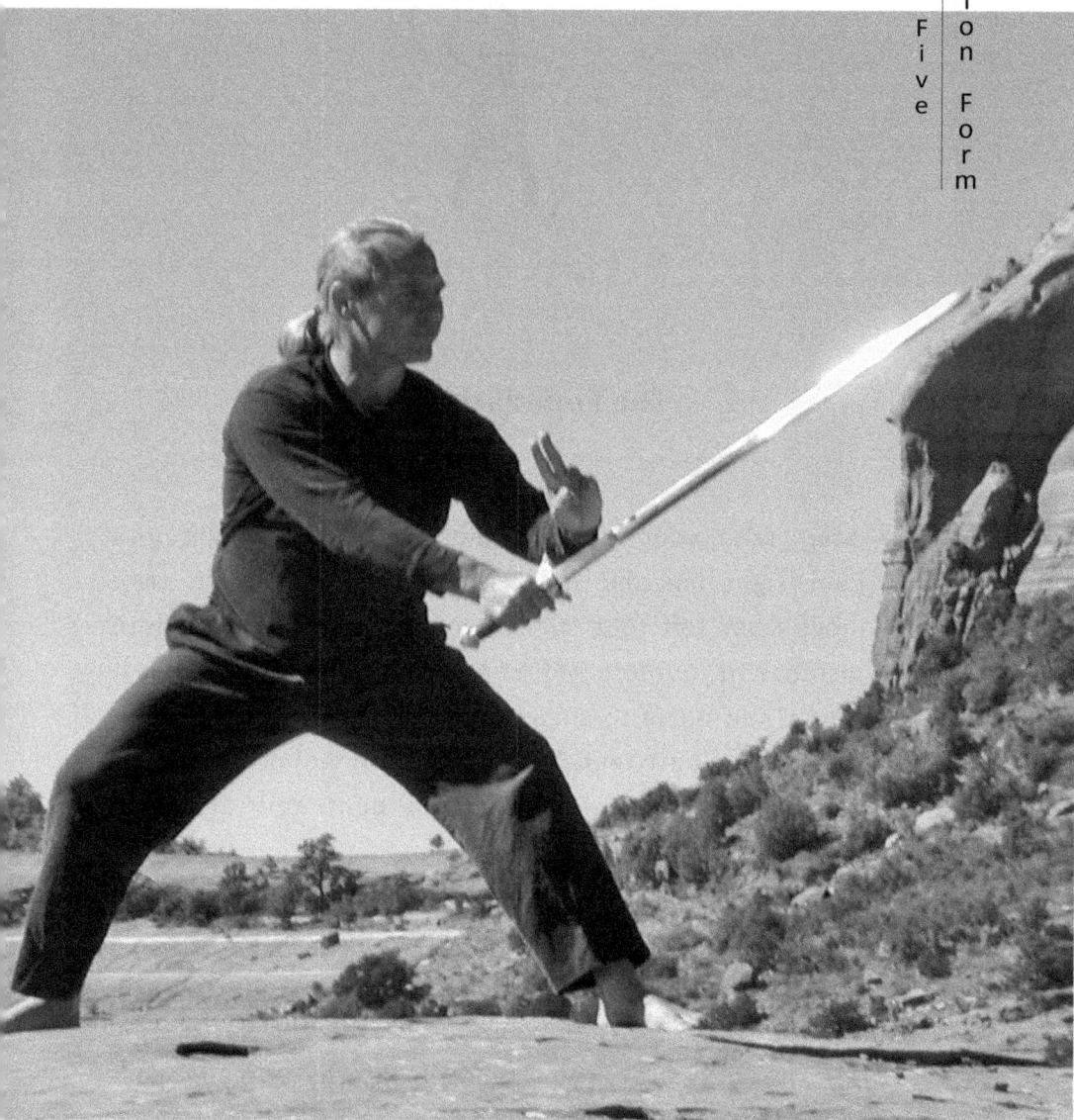

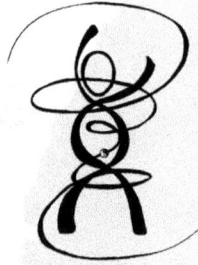

The Foundation Form

Opening

- Start with your feet together. Sink your weight into your right leg and foot, which frees your left. Now move your left foot slightly more than shoulder width distance to your left. At first place no weight into your left foot. Then move to the center, distributing your weight equally into both feet. The toes of both feet point straight ahead and your knees are slightly bent. Your arms and hands are completely relaxed, dangling at your sides.

- Form your Standing Posture, remembering the six adjustments ~ string, chin tuck, sink-fold-release, separated knees, knees bent, toes grab the earth. Feel the heaviness of your relaxed internal organs pass down through your released low back, sacrum, and tailbone into your feet. At the same time feel your spine lengthening through the top of your head. The tip of your tongue touches the roof of your mouth.

1. Draw Earth Qi

- Extend both arms forward and approximately 30° to the sides. Your hands are just below belly button height with the palms facing down. Your elbows are in front of your body, slightly bent, with the tips of your elbows pointing down (they are closer together than your wrists).

- Slightly flex your wrists so your palms literally face the earth and keep your hands aligned with your forearms.

- Extend and spread your fingers and thumbs in order to open your palms.

- Hold this position for two minutes.

2. Three Part Rise, Three Part Sink

- Without lifting your arms, move them to shoulder width and release your wrists. Your elbows are slightly bent with the tips of your elbows still pointing down. Remember to internally extend through your arms, hands and fingers while feeling the downward heaviness in your shoulders and elbows. Also feel the flexible strength in your wrists.

- Rise on your inhale, using the opening action of your

internal pumps. Your extended arms will be lifted to approximately shoulder height.

- Sink on your exhale, using the closing action of your internal pumps. Your arms will continue up to head height.

- Then rise again on your inhale. Your arms will extend to their highest point above your head. Keep your shoulders, elbows and wrists relaxed; your elbow tips are now pointing forward.

- Now sink on your exhale, using your internal pumps. As your extended arms are being lowered to approximately shoulder height, your wrist will flex allowing your hands and fingers to flow from the ends of your lowering arms.

- Rise on your inhale. You will continue to lower your arms to belly button height.

- Then sink again on your exhale, lowering your arms and hands to the level of your lower thighs.

- Do this complete movement two times.

3. Whirling Arms
- Completely release both arms and hands. You are now crouched with your arms dangling at your sides. Your hands are about knee height.

- Now rise abruptly. This feels like you are jumping straight up, though your feet remain on the earth. Allow the upward power of your internal pumps to propel your relaxed and yet extended arms and hands through the arc in front of your body that starts with your hands at your knees and finishes with your arms and hands extended above your head. At about the midpoint of this arc your wrists will briefly cross.

- Now sink abruptly. Allow the downward power of your pumps to pull your relaxed and yet extended arms and hands down through the arc behind your body that starts with your arms and hands extended above your head and ends with your hands at your knees.

- Whirl your arms 4 times in this direction.

- Now reverse direction. As you rise abruptly, guide your relaxed yet extended arms and hands upward through the arc behind your body. This arc ends with your arms and hands extended above your head.

- Then sink abruptly, guiding your relaxed yet extended arms and hands downward through the arc in front of your body. This arc ends with your hands again at your knees. At about the midpoint of this arc your wrists will briefly cross.

- Whirl your arms 4 times in this direction. Finish the last cycle when your wrists cross in front of your body at approximately chest height.

4. Embracing the Qi Ball of the Heart

- Your wrists will now uncross as you extend your arms and hands straight out from your body. Rotate your arms and hands so that your palms are now facing one another with about 15 inches between them. Your middle fingers are at nipple height.

- Slightly bend your elbows and wrists to form a roundness, as if you were embracing the field of energy emanating out from your Middle Tan Tien. Extend and spread your fingers and thumbs in order to open the palms. The center of each palm is now facing toward and communicating with the mid chest point between your breasts. The tips of your two middle fingers are 8-10 inches apart and complete the qi ball.

- This is a great time to recheck your Standing Posture. Go through the six adjustments ~ string, chin tuck, sink-fold-release, separated knees, knees bent, toes grab the earth. Feel the heaviness of your relaxed internal organs passing down through your released low back, sacrum and tailbone into your feet. At the same time feel your spine lengthening through the top of your head. The tip of your tongue touches the roof of your mouth.

- Hold this posture for two minutes.

5. Circle of the Four Expressions

- Sink slightly while walking your feet out to form a medium wide Horse Stance. The insides edges of your feet are now shoulder width apart and your knees are a little more bent.

- To start this movement, push from your left foot. This will move your body to the right. As you are moving right, also turn your legs and pelvis (the Lower Tan Tien) and your spine and chest (the Middle Tan Tien) to the right to their natural stopping points. As you are turning, move your extended and spiraling arms to the right as well. At the end of your turn, both arms are extended out to your side at shoulder height. Your right open palm is facing down; your left is facing up. Your left hand is even with your right elbow crease and approximately 4 inches from it. Remember to watch your lead right hand.

- Now push from your right foot, which moves your body to the left and also turns your Lower and Middle Tan Tiens to the left to their natural stopping points. Feel the internal heaviness of your relaxed organs and released low back, sacrum, and tailbone merging with the rising "push force" of your leg. Remember you are using the resulting peng force to contract your spine, close your chest, and turn your tan tiens. Use these internal movements of your body to draw down and spiral your extended arms and hands through an arc that passes just in front of your upper thighs. The spiraling within your arms and hands turns your palms to face down and diagonally forward; your hands and fingers are trailing behind your wrists. Watch your lead left hand. Your left finishes ten inches out to the side of your left upper thigh, your right following 15 inches behind.

- Now push from your left foot, which moves your body to the right and also turns your Lower and Middle Tan Tiens to the right to their natural stopping points. Feel again the internal heaviness of your relaxed organs and released low back, sacrum, and tailbone merging with the "rising-push force" of your leg. This time you are using the resulting peng force to lengthen your spine, expand your chest, and turn your tan tiens. Use these internal movements of your body to drive upward and spiral your extended arms and hands through an arc that passes in front of your forehead at top-of-head height. The spiraling in your arms and hands turns your palms to face forward and diagonally upward; your hands and fingers are trailing behind your wrists. Watch your lead right hand. Your right finishes about 12 inches out to the right side of your head, your left following approximately 18 inches behind.

- Then push from your right foot, which moves your body to the left and turns your Lower and Middle Tan Tiens to the left to their natural stopping points. You will again be using the peng force to turn your tan tiens. You will also use this force to contract your spine and close your chest through the first half of your turning, and then lengthen your spine and open your chest through the latter half of your turning. In the first half, these internal movements draw your extended arms and hands down through an arc that passes in front of your chest. Your palms are turning to face down and diagonally forward. In the later half, your internal movements propel and spiral your arms and hands through a push to your left side. At the end of the push, both palms are pressing out to your left side at chest height, fingers pointing forward. Your hands are about 12 inches apart.

• You will now move through the three phases of this movement in the reverse direction – pushing from your left foot to draw your arms and hands down to the right, pushing from your right foot to drive your arms and hands upward to the left, and finally pushing from your left foot to propel your arms and hands through the push to the right at chest height.

• Do four complete cycles, finishing in the palm-push to the right side at chest height.

6. Spiral Open, Spiral Close

• Come back to center position, distributing your weight equally in both feet. Release your arms, allowing them to dangle at your sides. You are still in a medium wide Horse Stance.

(The leg and body movements in Spiral Open, Spiral Close

are the same as the previous movement. It is only the arm and hand movements that change.)

- Push from your right foot. This will move your body to the left and at the same time turn your Lower and Middle Tan Tiens to the left to their natural stopping points. Both downwardly extended arms with extended fingers and thumbs begin to move to the left with your right arm passing under the left so that your wrists cross. Both arms and hands are spiraling so that the open palms are turning to face diagonally away from the body. You are now turned left with both arms extended down to your left, approximately 12 inches out from your thigh. The crossed wrists are at belly button height, and you are watching your lead, right hand.

- Now push from your left foot. As your body is moving to the right, you are at the same time turning your Lower and Middle Tan Tiens to the right. Here you must use your peng force to drive the three body movements of lengthening your spine, opening the chest, and turning the legs and pelvis and the spine and chest. These three body movements lift your elbows to shoulder hight. At this point, your forearms are relaxed and your crossed wrists are about 4 inches out from the mid-chest point. The spiraling arms continue rising through your left side with your wrists uncrossing. At about the mid point of your turning, both arms are extended above your head, and your arms and hands have continued to spiral so that the open palms now face upward. At the end of your turn to the right, when the tan tiens have reached their natural stopping points, both arms are extended out to their perspective sides at shoulder height. The open palms are facing away from your body, fingers pointing up. You are watching your lead, right hand.

- Then push from your right foot. This moves your body to the left, though this time you will stop in the center. You are at the same time turning your Lower and Middle Tan Tiens to the left, but they, too, will stop at the center when your pelvis and chest are facing forward. Here you must again use your peng force to drive the three body movements of contracting your spine, closing the chest, and turning your legs and pelvis (Lower Tan Tien) and spine and chest (Middle Tan Tien). The turning of your tan tiens along with the contraction of your spine and the closing of your chest draws and spirals your elbows down and in toward your body. This action also causes both hands to grab, starting with your little fingers and continuing with your ring, middle, index, and thumbs. With this spiraling action, pull the Qi into your Lower Tan Tien. You finish facing forward with both fists touching your lower abdomen. The spiraling action in your arms has turned your hands so that the palm side of your fists face up.

- Relax your arms and hands, allowing them to dangle at your sides to begin the next move.

- Do this movement 4 times to the left and 4 times in the reverse direction.

- You will finish facing forward with both upward turned fists touching your lower abdomen 2 inches below your belly button.

7. Drawing Qi From Heaven

- Open both fists, extending and spreading your fingers and thumbs to open your palms. Both palms are now facing up, fingers pointing toward one another with approximately 2 inches separating the middle fingers. Your elbows move slightly forward so the elbow tips point out to the sides.

- As you inhale, rise. Lift both hands up the front of your body to the level of your forehead while keeping your palms turned upward. In front of your forehead, rotate both hands almost 360° so the open palms again face the sky.

- Slightly sink while releasing your low back, sacrum, and tailbone into the earth. At the same time, extend your spiraling arms and hands to press your palms toward heaven. This position is like hitting a volleyball with your palms and fingers. Slightly elevate your chin to look upward through the triangle formed by your thumbs and index fingers.

- Hold this position for one minute.

8. Striking with Open Palms

- Lower both upward facing palms down the front of your body to breast height. This happens with a continuous spiraling motion that's like lowering two cups of tea from heaven. When your hands reach the chest, your open palms are still facing up with the little finger sides of both your hands resting lightly against your body just below your breasts. Draw your elbows slightly back and in against your body. Your extended fingers now point diagonally forward toward the midline.

- Push from your left foot. As your body moves to the right and your tan tiens begin turning to the right, pivot your right foot on its heel until your toes point 45° to the right.

- Bend your right knee as you transfer all of your weight into your right leg. Then drawn in your left foot placing it 3 inches to the left of your right. At this point, your left carries no weight and only the ball of the foot is touching the ground. Your pelvis, chest, and head are also facing 45° to the right.

- Allow the weight of your body passing down through your released low-back, sacrum, and tailbone, to root you into your right leg as you now extend your left foot straight forward with the toes also pointing forward. Place no weight into your left, though the entire sole is touching the earth. Remember to maintain the 3-inch channel running between your feet from front to back and keep your released tailbone in alignment with your back heel.

- At the same time that you are extending your foot, you also extend your left arm straight forward at breast height. The arm and hand are spiraling so that the open palm faces forward, fingers pointing up. Your elbow is slightly bent with the tip of your elbow pointing down. Also lower your right hand down the right side of your body to waist level. The open palm is facing up and the fingers are pointing forward. Your head turns to watch your left, lead hand, but your pelvis and chest are still facing 45° to the right.

- Push from your right, back foot; this moves your body forward. As you are moving forward, also turn your Lower and Middle Tan Tiens to the left until both your pelvis and chest are facing forward. They arrive to this position at the same time that your front, left knee comes to its stopping point just shy of the tips of your toes. The pushing (pumps 1, 2 and 3) and the turning of your tan tiens (pump 4) drive the heel of your right, open palm from its waist position along a direct path to become the forward extended arm and hand at breast height. The arm and hand are spiraling so that the open palm faces forward, fingers pointing up. Your elbow is slightly bent with the tip of your elbow pointing down. At the same time, the internal pumps are drawing your left hand from its extended position along a direct line to your waist at the left side of your body. The arm and hand are spiraling so that the open palm is facing up and the fingers are pointing forward.

- You watch your lead, right hand.

- Now push from your front, left foot. This moves your body back. As you are moving back, turn your Lower and Middle Tan Tiens to the right until both your pelvis and chest again face the 45°, right diagonal. At this point your released tailbone is aligned with and pointing down to your back, right heel. The pushing and turning drive the heel of your left, open plam from its waist position directly forward to become the forward extended arm and hand at breast height. The arm and hand are spiraling so that the open palm faces forward, fingers pointing up. Remember that the elbow is slightly bent with the tip pointing down. Your right hand is drawn from its extended position directly back to your waist at the right side of your body. The spiraling action in your arm turns your hand so that the palm faces up, fingers pointing forward.

- You watch your lead, left hand.

- Do this forward-back movement four times, finishing in the back position.

- Now change sides. Being deeply rooted in your right leg and foot, draw your left foot in adjacent to your right. Then extend it behind you and 3 inches to the left in order to maintain your channel. The entire foot touches the ground, though you place no weight into it. The toes point 45° to the left. Then push from your right foot; this moves your body back and transfers your weight into your left foot. Your Lower and Middle Tan Tiens will turn so that your pelvis and chest face the 45°, left diagonal. Lastly, your right foot needs to pivot slightly on the heel so that the toes point forward.

• The push from your front, right leg and the turning of your tan tiens to the left again drive your right spiraling arm and hand from the palm-up-waist-position directly to the palm-out-extended-position, and draw your spiraling left arm and hand from the palm-out-extended-position directly to the palm-up-waist-position. Your released tailbone is now aligned with and pointing down to your back, left heel.

• You watch your lead, right hand.

• You are now set to do the forward-back movement four more times on this side. Finish in the back position, right arm extended and left hand at your waist.

9. Grabbing The Tree's Qi
• Allow the heaviness of your organs to pass through your released low back, sacrum and tailbone into your back, left leg and turn your pelvis and chest a little more left. At the same time release your arms and

hands, allowing them to fall in front of your thighs.

- Now push from your back, left leg. As your body moves forward, turn your Lower and Middle Tan Tiens to also face forward. Allow the push from your leg and the turning of your tan tiens to lift both elbows up the front of your body. Your forearms, wrists and hands remain completely relaxed as your rising elbows drag them up the front of your abdomen until your thumbs are at breast height.

- When your thumbs reach breast height, you are at the halfway point in both the forward movement of your body and the turning of your tan tiens.

- As you continue to push forward and turn your pelvis and chest to face forward, your arms and hands then engage to travel in an upward and forward arc. Your arms and hands are spiraling so that your palms, which were facing down, now are turning to face forward.

- Your pelvis and chest come to their forward facing position at the same time that your front, right knee arrives at its stopping point. Remember to never drive your knee past your toes. Your arms and hands are reaching forward with your hands at hairline height. The spiraling in your arms has turned your open palms with extended fingers and thumbs to face forward. Your fingers are pointing diagonally up toward the centerline. The tips of your index fingers are about

4 inches apart. You feel like you are reaching out to grab a tree's Qi.

- You are watching your lead, right hand.

- Now push from your front, right leg. As your body moves back, turn your Lower and Middle Tan Tiens to face the 45°, left diagonal. Allow the push from your leg and the turning of your tan tiens to pull your elbows down and in toward the body. This spiraling action causes both hands to grab, starting with the little fingers and continuing through your ring, middle, index and thumbs. You use these spirals in your arms and hands to pull the Qi into your lower abdomen.

- You finish the movement with 90% of your weight on the back leg and with your relaxed tailbone aligned with and pointing down to your back, left heel. Your pelvis and chest are facing the 45°, left diagonal. Both fists are touching your lower abdomen. The spiraling action in your arms turns your hands so that the palm side of your fists face up.

- You are watching your lead, left hand.

- As you begin the next push from your back, left leg, relax your wrists and hands as your rising elbows again drag your forearms and hands up the front of your abdomen.

- Repeat the movement four times, finishing in the back position.

- To change sides, you again push from your back, left leg. But this time you use the forward movement of your body and the turning of your tan tiens to pivot your forward, right foot so that the toes point 45° to the right. As this happens, your rising elbows are dragging your relaxed forearms, wrists and hands up the front of your abdomen until the thumbs are at breast height. Then push from your right foot as you step forward with your left. Commit your weight to your now forward, left foot. Remember to step with a 3-inch channel and have your toes point straight ahead. As this happens, your arms and hands are engaging to travel in their upward, forward arc. You finish with your weight forward and your pelvis and chest facing forward. Your arms and hands are reaching forward with your open palms facing forward. Your hands are at hairline height. You again feel like you are reaching out to grab the tree's Qi.

- Push from your front, left foot, which moves your body back and turns your Lower and Middle Tan Tiens to face the 45°, right diagonal. These internal movements again pull your elbows down and in toward the body. The spiraling action in your arms and hands is what grabs and pulls the Qi into your lower abdomen.

- Repeat Grabbing the Tree's Qi 4 more times on this side, finishing in the back position.

- Draw your left foot in next to your right. Transfer your weight into your left foot which frees your right to step out into a slightly wider than shoulder width stance. Now center your weight. Sink slightly and release your arms and hands, allowing them to dangle in front of your thighs.

Close

- Internally extend through your arms, hands, and fingers while keeping your shoulders, elbows, and wrists relaxed. Your arms and hands are shoulder width apart, palms facing back.

- Rise on your inhalation. As you rise, use the opening action of your internal pumps to lift your extended arms, hands, and fingers up to breast height. Remember to keep your elbow tips pointing down and remember how your hands and fingers flow behind your wrists. Then continue to use your rise and expanding chest to further carry your extended arms up and out to your sides. At this point you are fully risen and your extended and yet relaxed arms are spread out to your sides like wings. The tops of your wrists are approximately 8 inches above shoulder height with your open palms facing down. Now extend your fingers and thumbs so that they feel like the long prongs of a pitchfork.

- Sink on your exhalation. Use the closing action of your internal pumps to drive your extended arms and your long fingers down through your sides and into the earth. This feels like you are plunging your energy fingers deep into the earth to gather her Qi. At this point you are sunk down with your wrists just below knee height. Your open palms are shoulder width apart and facing one another. The extended fingers are pointing diagonally down.

- Rise on your inhalation. Use the opening action of your pumps to lift your up-turned palms to solar plexus height. This feels like you are lifting the earth's Qi up into your body. At this point you are fully risen. Your palms are facing up at the solar plexus with your extended fingers pointing towards one another. The tips of your middle fingers are 1 inch apart.

- On your exhalation, abruptly sink and abruptly drop your up-turned palms to the level of your pelvic floor. This feels like you have dropped four grocery bags of earth into your pelvis. This sudden release drives your Qi into your tailbone in order that it can travel up your spine.

- Rise on your inhalation. Again use the opening action of your pumps to lift your extended arms through your sides. Your arms are spiraling which turns your open palms to first face forward and then upward as they continue to rise through their arcs. At this point you are fully risen with both arms and hands extended above your head. Your open palms are facing one another, shoulder width apart, fingers pointing up. The intention in this movement is to bring the Qi up your spine to the top of your head.

- While still inhaling, do a slight but abrupt sink and rise. As you sink, your extended arms move out to your sides and forward in a circular, gathering motion. Your arms spiral, which turns your open palms to face forward and then face one another. This movement is the outward, reaching part of the gathering. As you rise, you complete the gathering by drawing your extended arms back towards you. The arms continue to spiral, turning your open palms to face back. This movement is the inward, collecting part of the gathering. At this point, you are fully risen with both arms extended above your head. Your elbows are slightly bent with the tips of your elbows pointing forward. Your open palms are facing back, fingers pointing up. Your hands are 3 inches apart. The intention in this movement is to gather the Qi of heaven into your head.

- Now extend and spread your fingers and thumbs to open your palms and bring your awareness into your palms. Sink as you exhale. As you sink, draw your palms down the front of your face and throat to the heart point between your breasts. At this level your elbows will move slightly out to your sides. Do not rise or sink and keep your palms facing your chest as you lift your elbows so that your fingers now point down. Continue to exhale as you now rise. As you rise, continue moving your open palms down the front of your body all the way to your lower abdomen (2 inches below your belly button). This movement brings the Qi down the front of your body, returning it to "The Sea of Qi," your Lower Tan Tien.

- Hold this position for a while with the intention of nurturing yourself.

- Keep your awareness in your Lower Tan Tien as you move your hands away from your lower abdomen. Then release you arms and hands, allowing them to dangle at your sides. Draw your left foot in adjacent to your right.

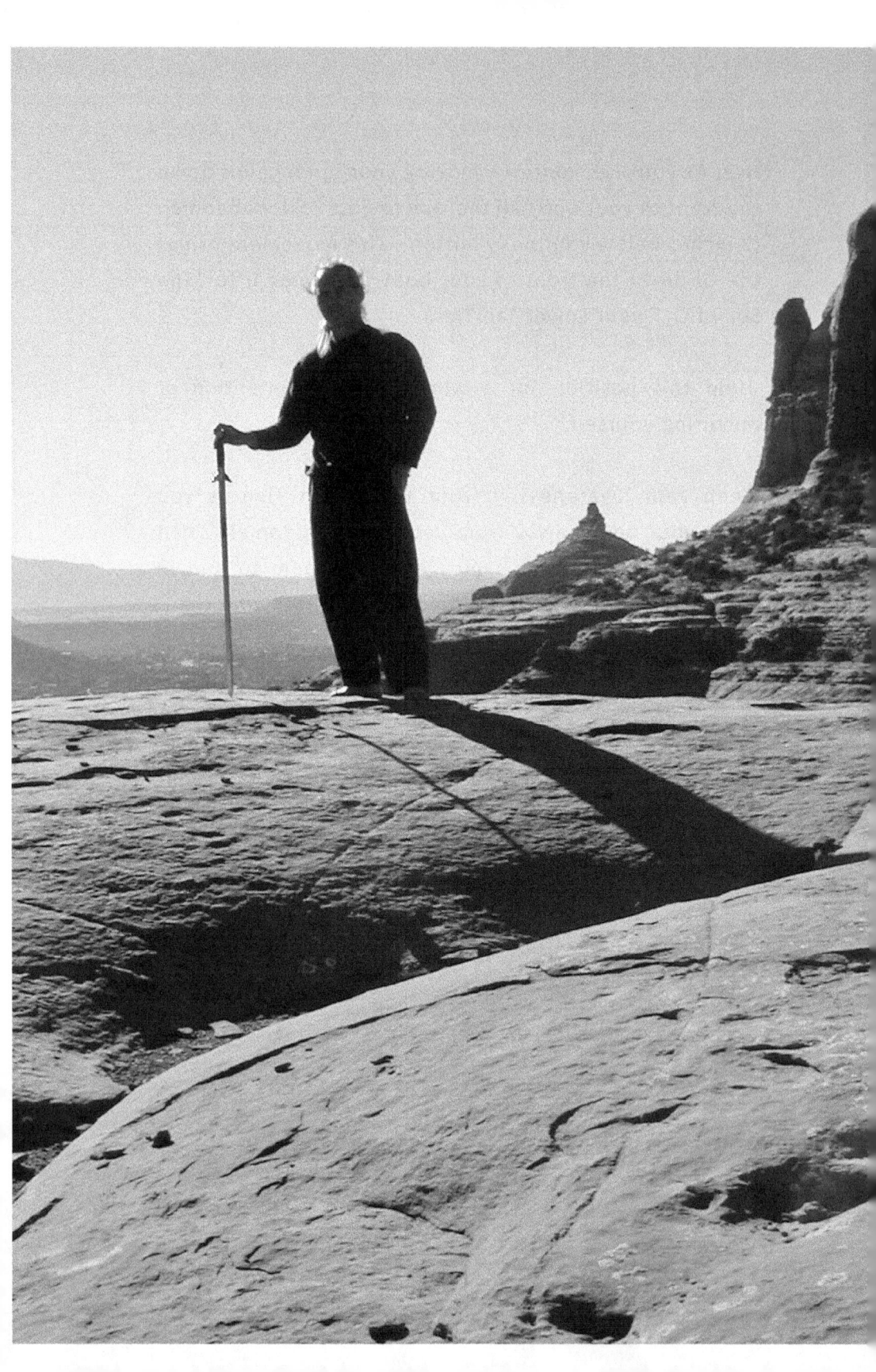

About the Author

Lyn Dilbeck is a thirty-year practitioner of Qi Gong and Internal Martial Arts. He currently lives in Sedona, Arizona where he has been teaching these arts for the past twenty years.

To know himself and to help others know themselves has always been the deepest motivating force in Lyn's life. This heart-felt desire is the essence of his Qi Gong Practice and what he shares as a teacher.

Before Lyn started to develop a conscious relationship with Qi through Qi Gong Practice, his quest had taken him into metaphysics and the practice of meditation. Also having a desire to help others, he studied and practiced medicine as a Pediatric and Internal Medicine Physicians Assistant. These earlier studies and life experiences helped him to see that the power and intelligence that give us health is what heals us when we are ill. He felt that this intelligent power must be what sustains every level of our existence ~ physical, energetic, emotional and mental, and it must be connected somehow to the life purpose within each of us.

For Lyn, accepting that health, healing and spirituality were interconnected, was an epiphany that changed the direction of his life. He decided to seek out this intelligent power, to know it within himself, and to help others to know it within themselves.

In the mid-seventies, many people seeking a physical/energetic practice based in spirituality were studying Yoga, Aikido or Tai Qi Chuan. Lyn studied all three forms, yet it was in the practice of the traditional Yang Style of Tai Qi Chuan that he experienced those first "tastes" of a force flowing in and around him.

Lyn has come to know Qi Gong Practice as a conscious conversation between human beings and the intelligent power of Creation, Qi. In the course of this conversation he has learned that Qi is the divine intelligence and power that is birthing God's infinite potential into Creation. This is her true gong (purpose), to be the Mother of all vibrational existence and our Mother as well.

Lyn has spent the majority of his life tending to this relationship, and been fortunate to study with many gifted masters of Qi Gong and Internal Martial Arts:
• Ralf Cahn, Albany, CA ~ Kang jo fu
• Stephen Labensart, Mt. Shasta, CA ~ Yang Style Tai Qi Chuan
• Lily Soux, Honolulu, HI ~ Qi Gong
• George Xu, San Francisco, CA ~ Chen Style Tai Qi Chuan

- Chris Luth, Solano Beach, CA ~ Push Hands Training
- Master Zhou Ting Jue, Los Angeles, CA ~ Qi Gong (Wu Dang Style), Tai Qi Chuan, Hsing I, Bagua
- Miranda Warburton, Flagstaff, AZ ~ Hsing I, Bagua
- Master Li Jun Feng, Austin, TX ~ Qi Gong (Sheng Zhen)
- Master Chris Petrilli, Sedona, AZ ~ Escrima

Passionate and generous in all that he shares; Lyn excels in revealing the internal principles of these arts through demonstration and metaphor. His deeper gift however, is the way he shows that these principles are the same keys that allow our true nature to manifest into our life as joy, wisdom, health and love.

In addition to his own practice and teaching, Lyn is a lover of nature. You can often find him on a lake or river, boating and camping. He loves Mexico where he has lived and traveled; he also teaches Spanish as a second language.

Please look for the next manual and DVD in the series:
Guiding Principles of the Internal Arts
An Instructional Manual for Qi Gong Practice

FOR MORE INFORMATION about these teachings, acquiring the instructional manuals and DVDs, Lyn's workshops, or hosting a workshop in your area, please contact Lyn via his website: www.spiralinglifeforce.com

www.ingramcontent.com/pod-product-compliance
Lightning Source LLC
Chambersburg PA
CBHW071744090426

42738CB00011B/2563